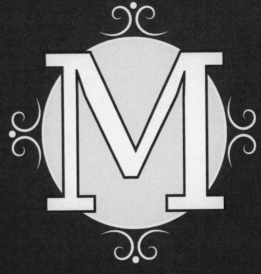

is for Medicine

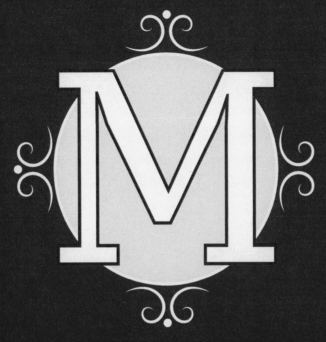

is for Medicine

by
Veronica Goodman

Illustrations by
Nicole Jones Sturk

For my Mom and Dr. Goodman

First Printing, 2019
ISBN 978-1-7320857-8-7

The images were created using vector design and the text was set in PT Serif Caption.

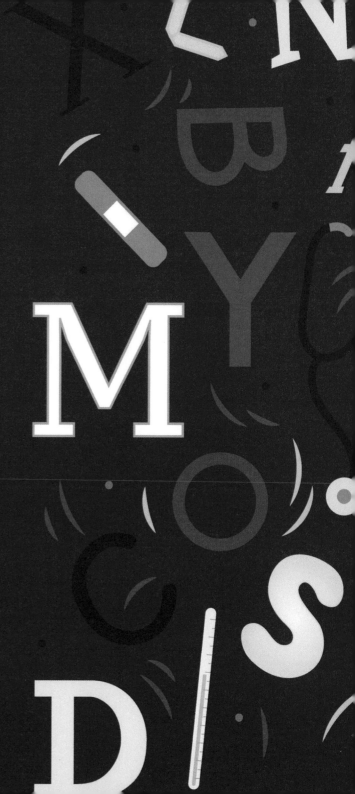

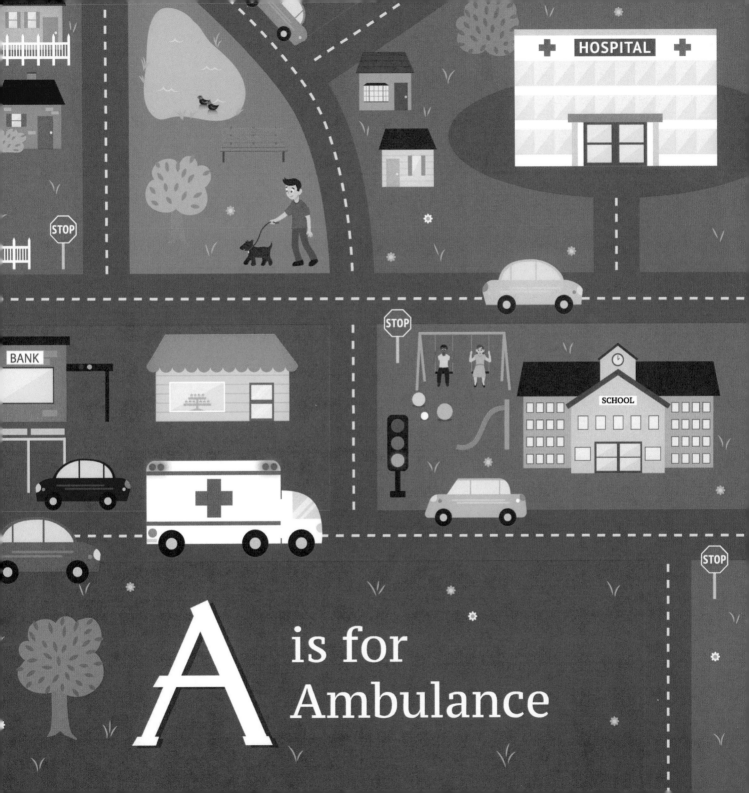

B
is for
Bandage

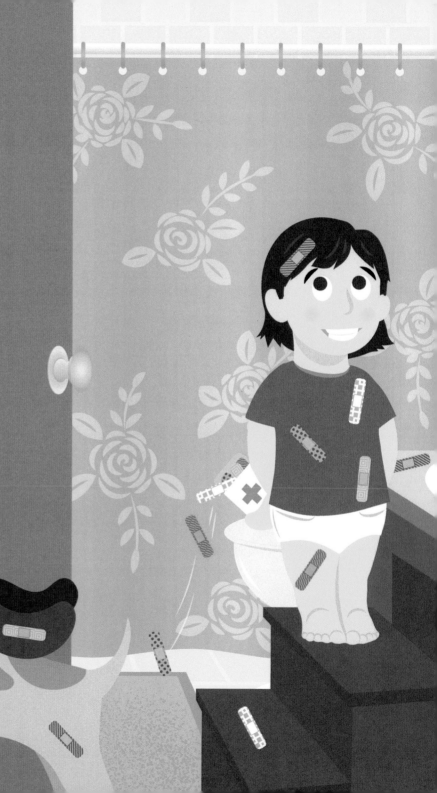

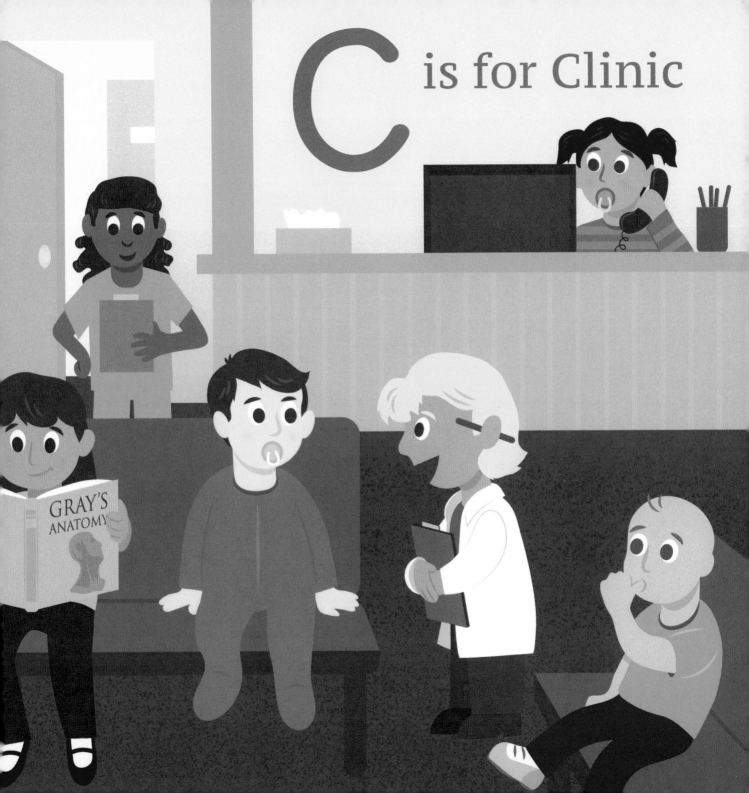

C is for Clinic

D is for Doctor

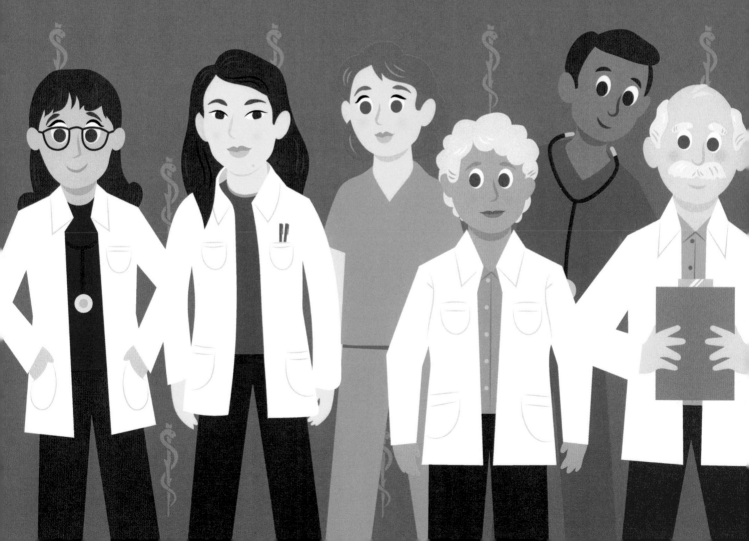

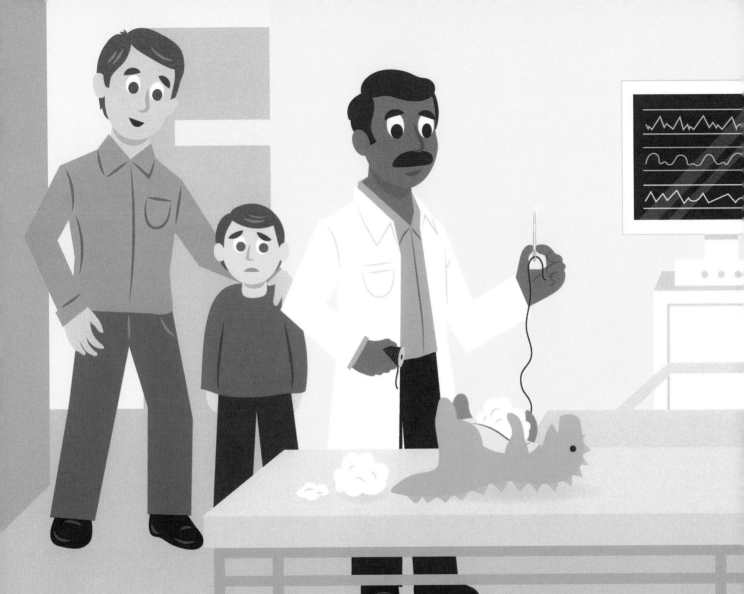

E is for
Emergency Room

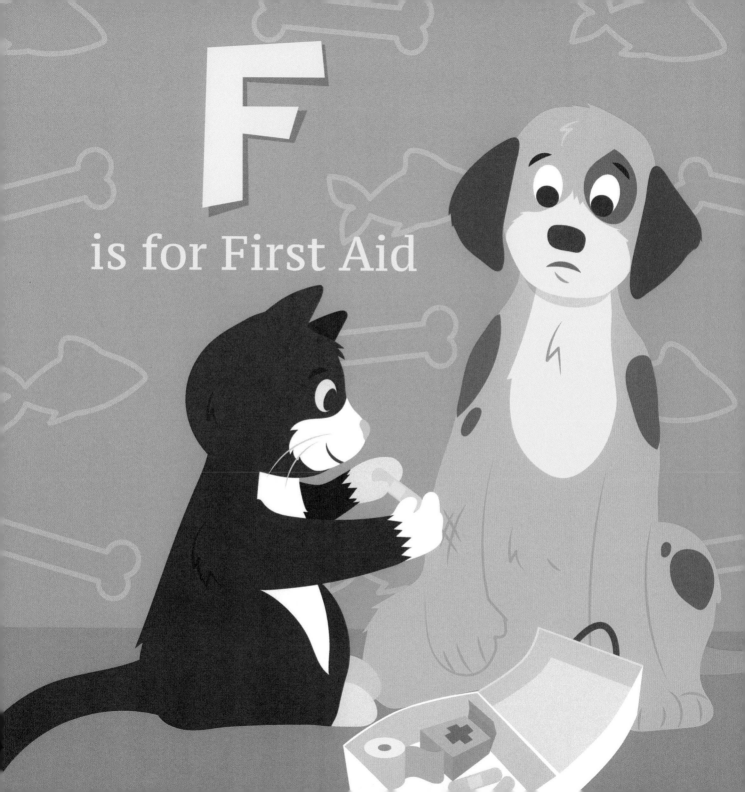

F
is for First Aid

G is for Genetics

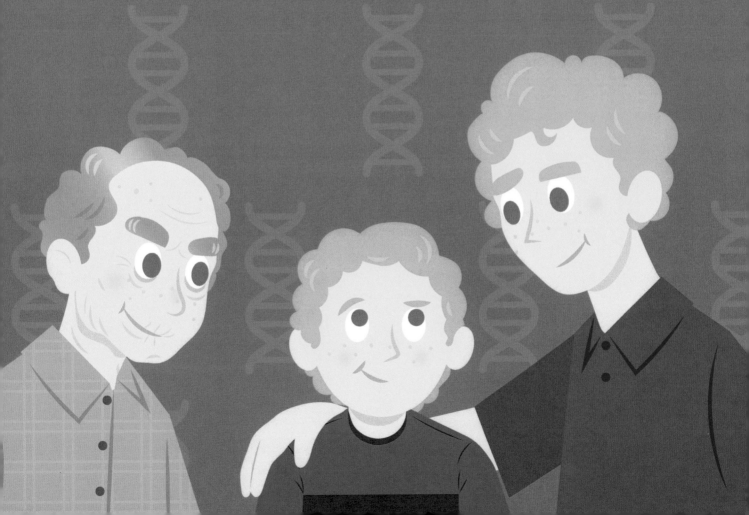

H

is for Hospital

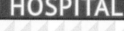

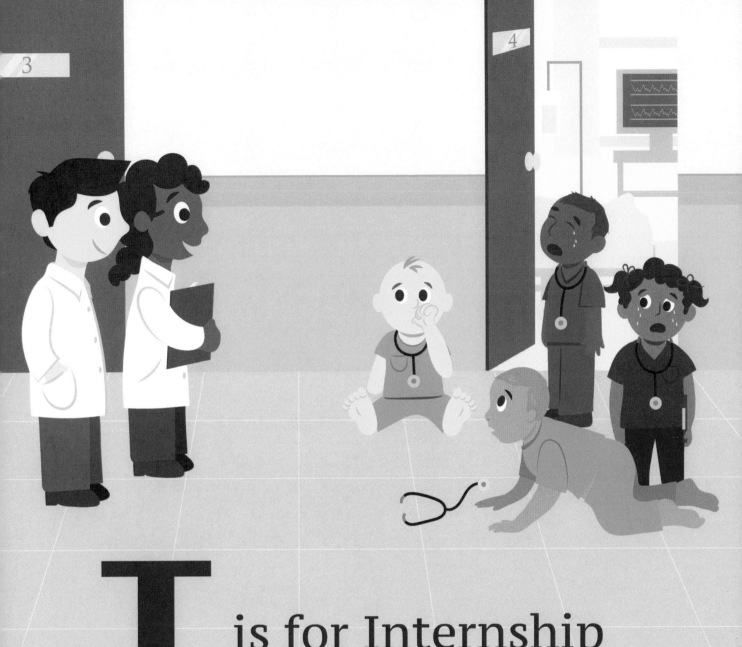

I is for Internship

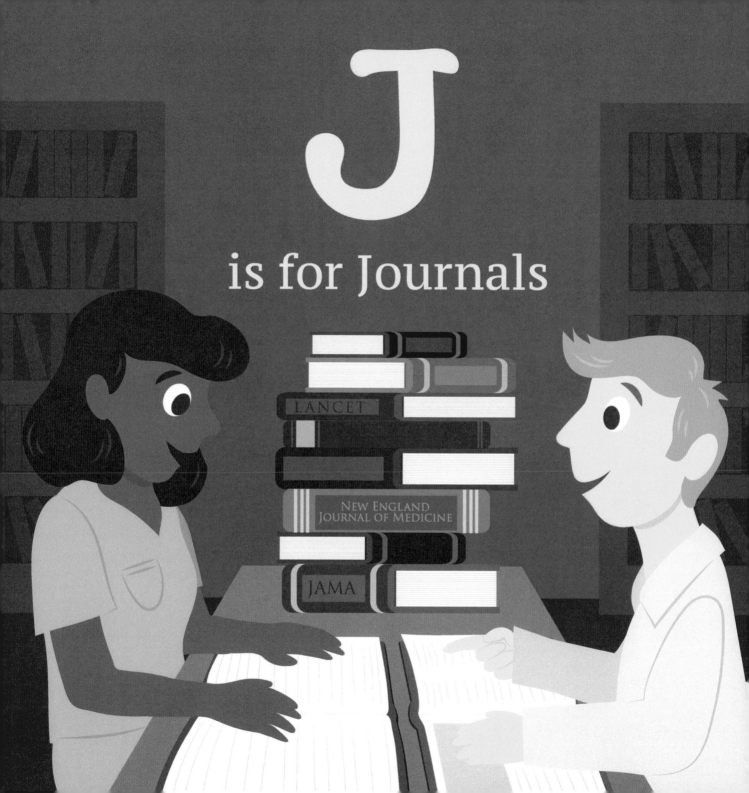

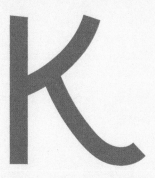

K

is for Keeping the Doctor Away

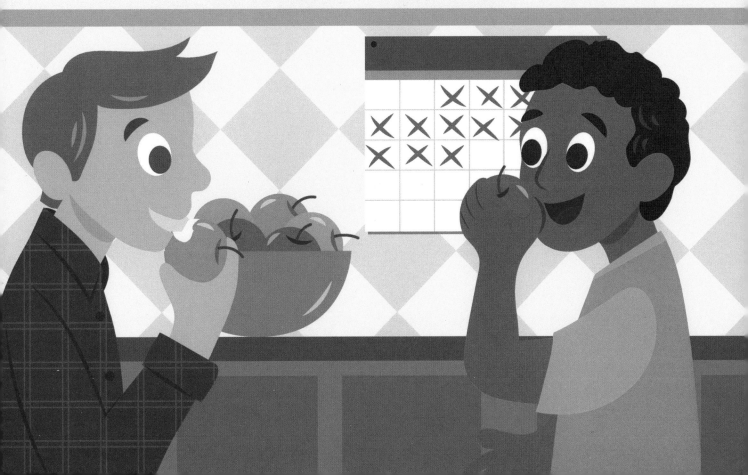

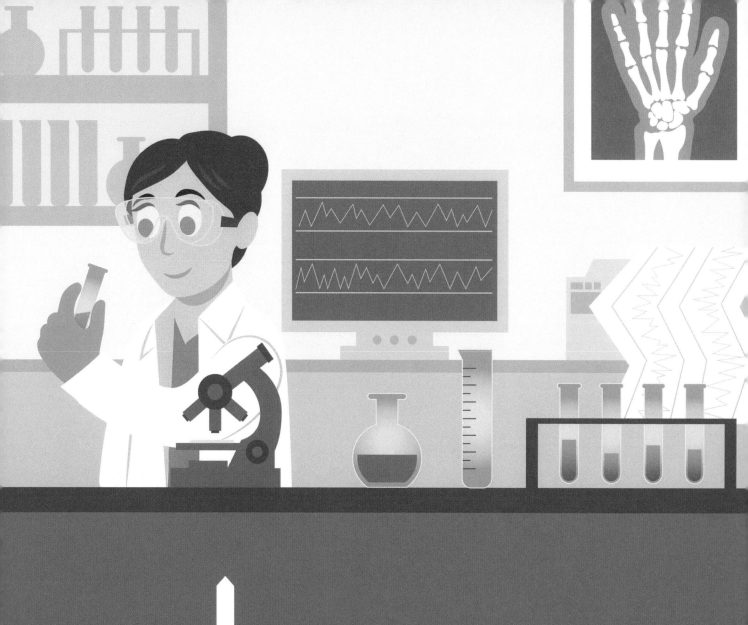

is for Labs

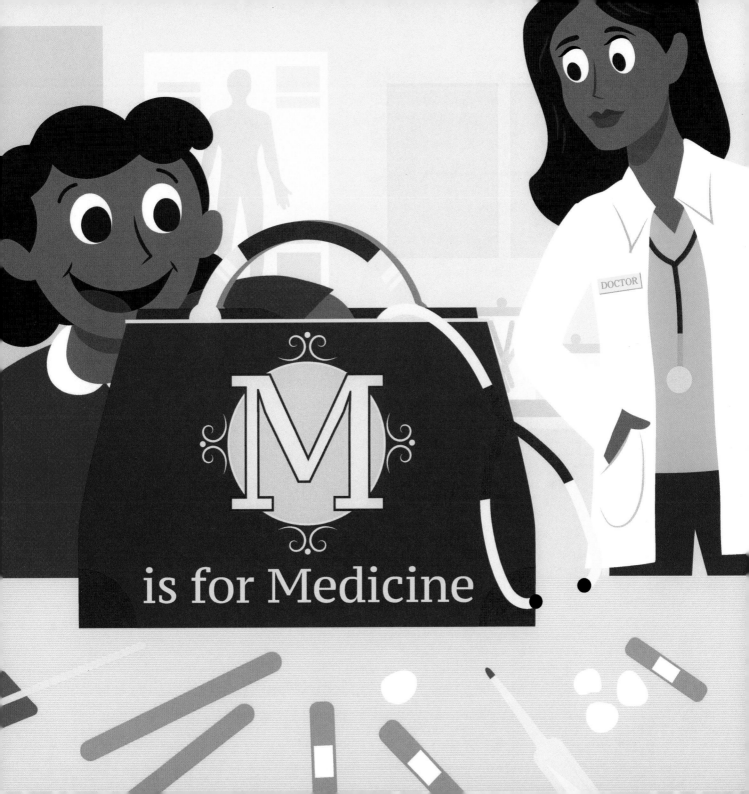

is for Medicine

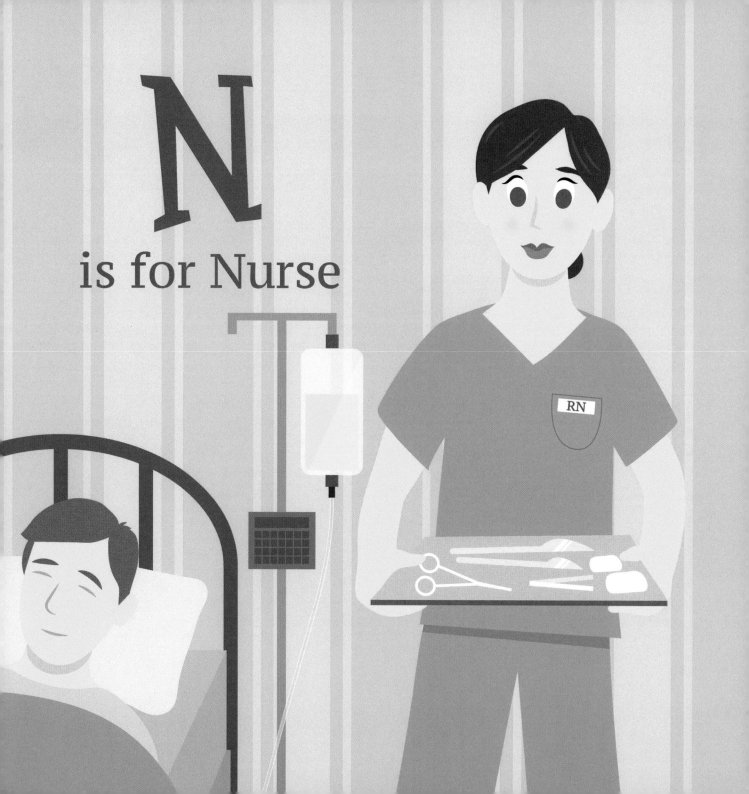

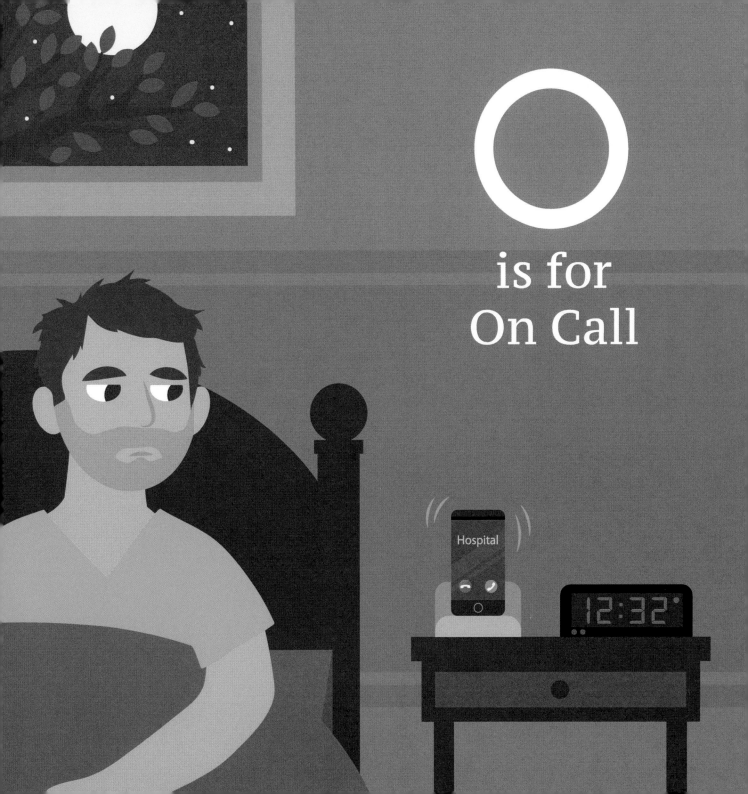

is for
On Call

P is for Patient

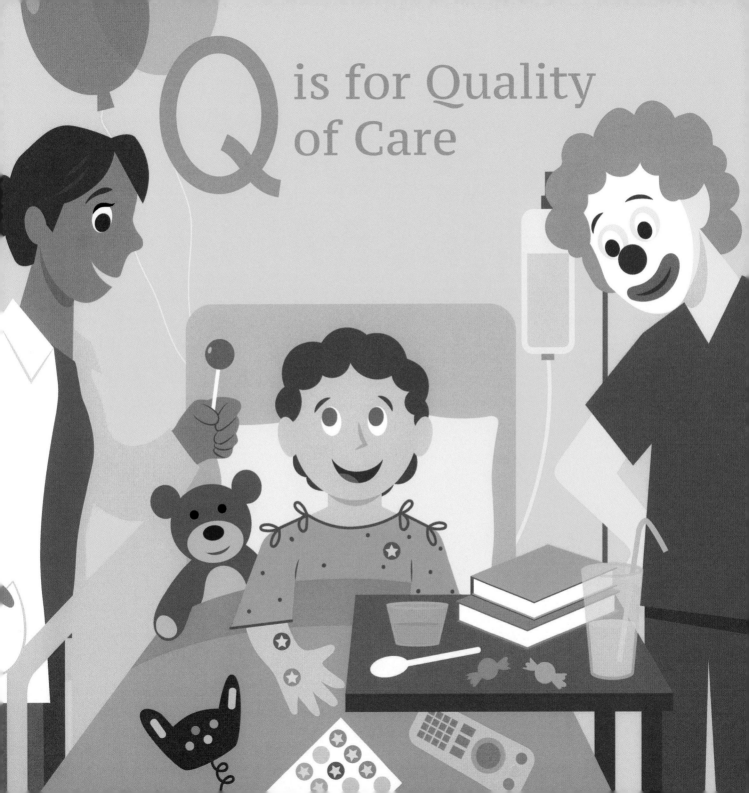

Q is for Quality of Care

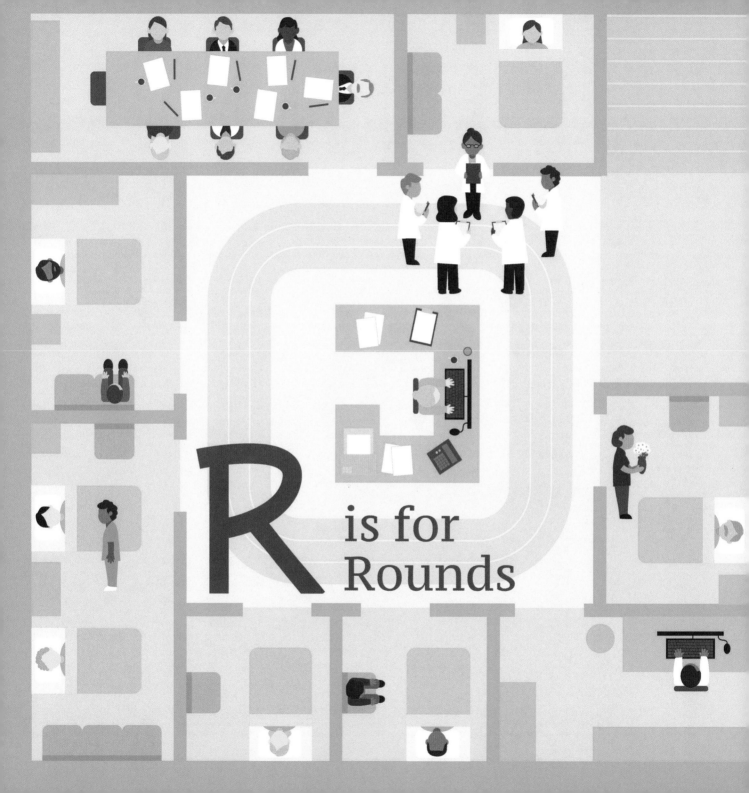

R is for
Rounds

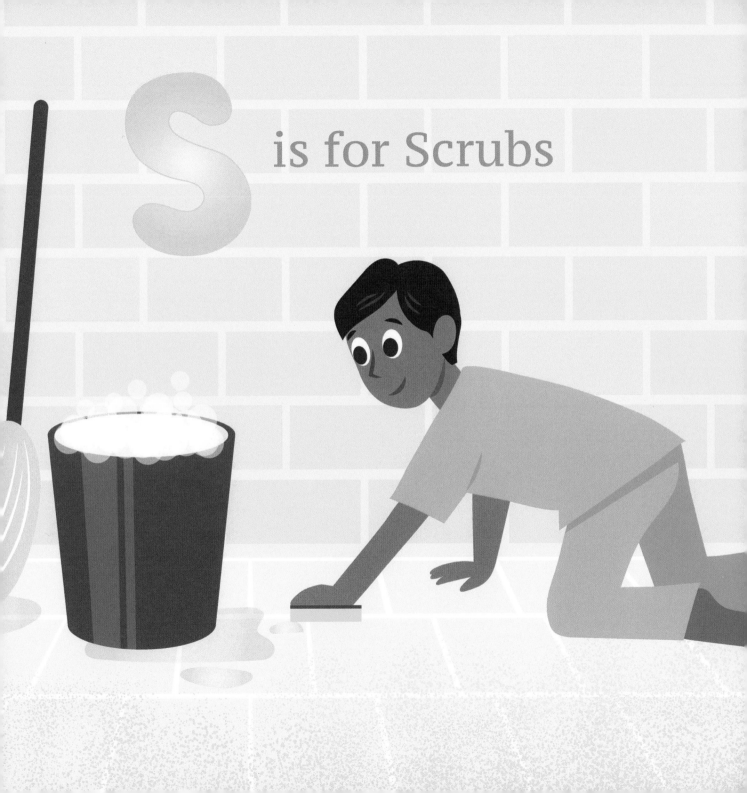

S is for Scrubs

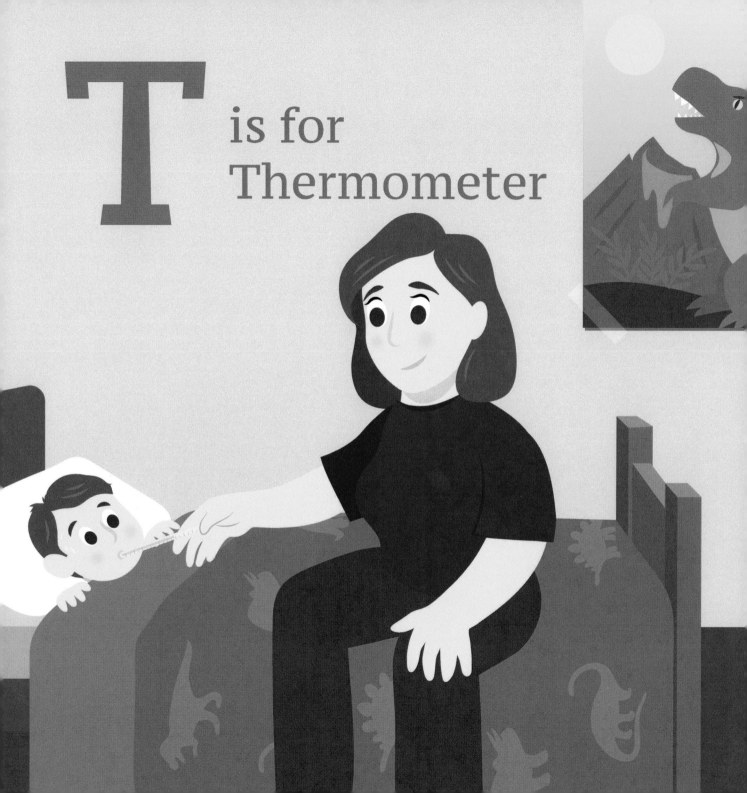

T

is for
Thermometer

U is for Ultrasound

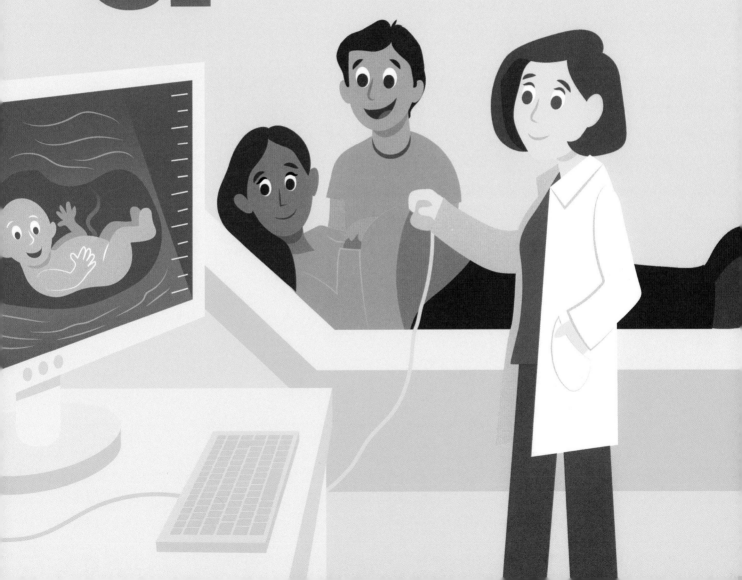

HR   bpm
60

SpO$_2$
99
%

Resp   rpm
18

118 / 70 BP

is for Vital Signs

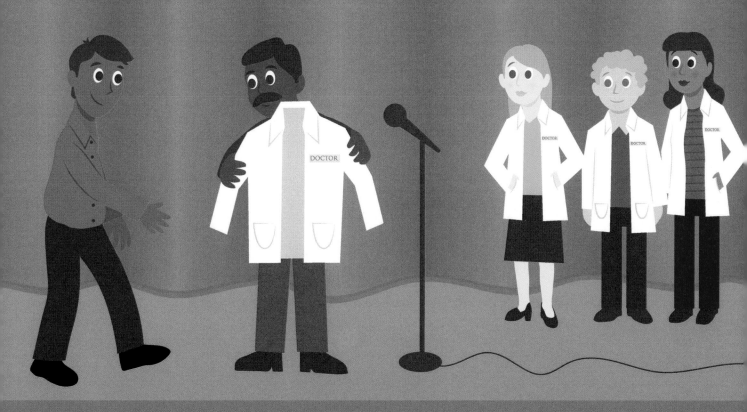

W is for White Coat

X is for X-ray

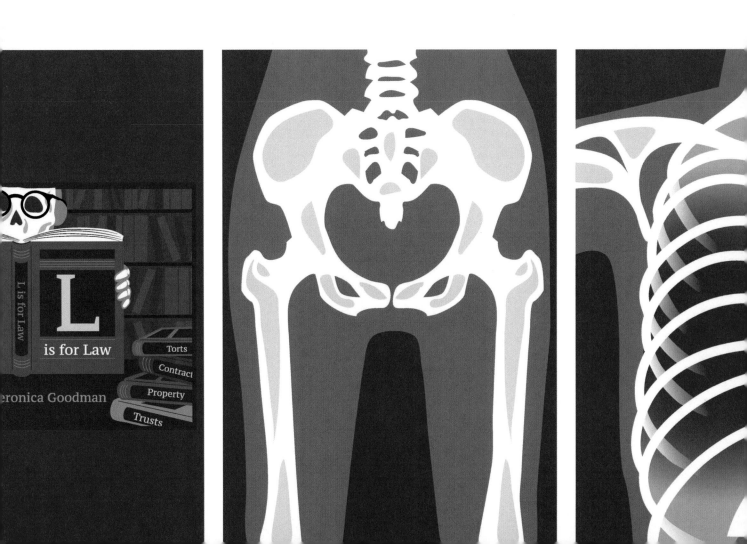

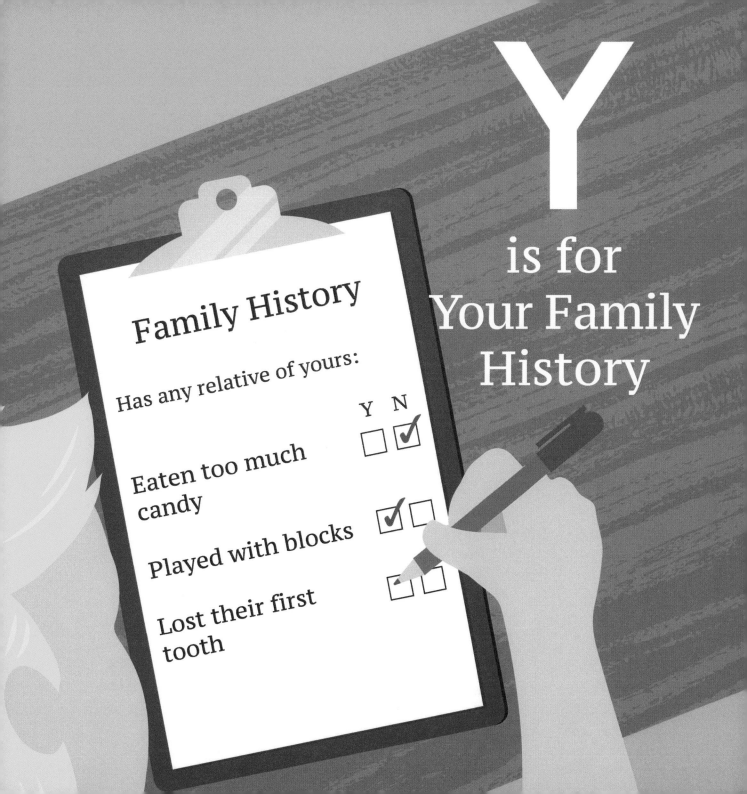

Y

is for
Your Family History

Family History

Has any relative of yours:

Y N

Eaten too much
candy

Played with blocks

Lost their first
tooth

Z

is for Zoom In

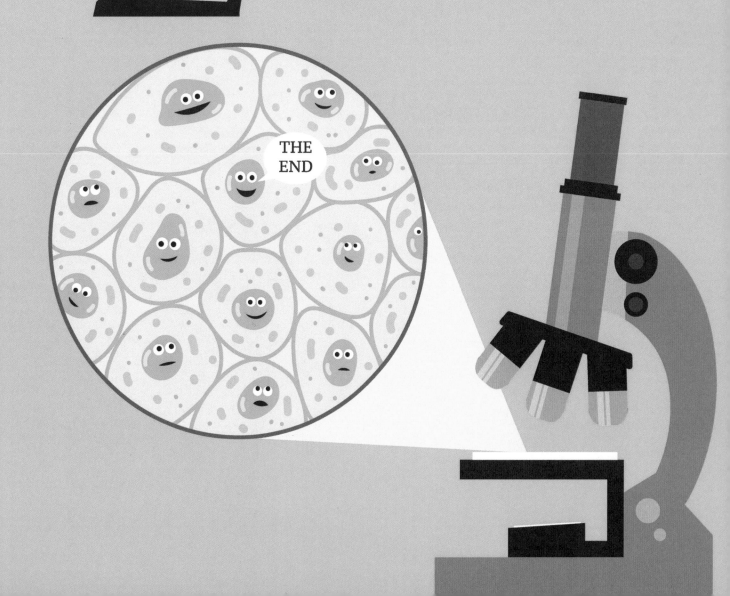

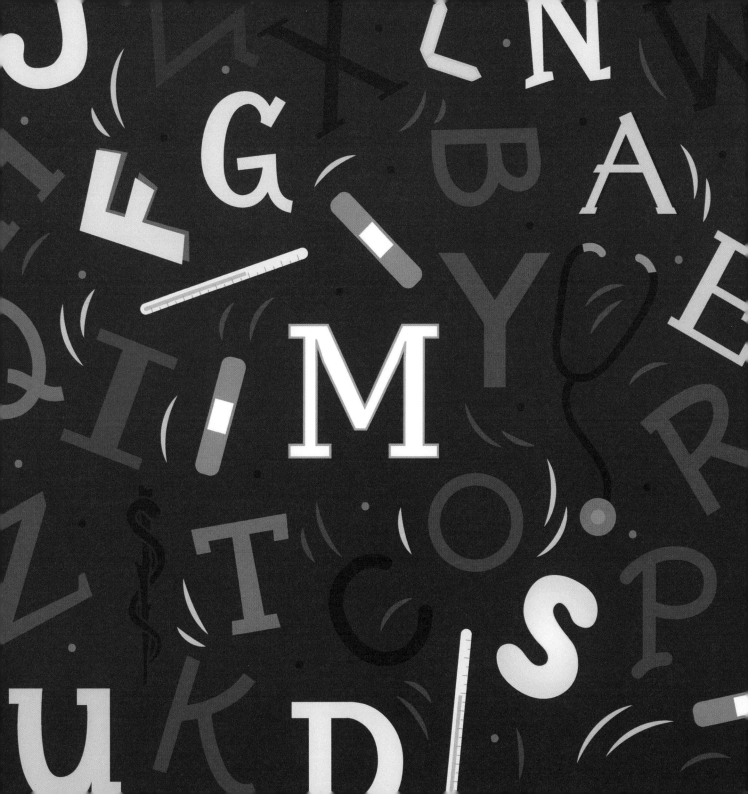